Copyright © 2026 by Joshua Moroles
All rights reserved.

No part of this book may be reproduced, stored in a retrieval system, or transmitted in any form or by any means electronic, mechanical, photocopying, recording, or otherwise without prior written permission of the publisher, except for brief quotations used in reviews or scholarly works.

This book is published by
Ryker Blueprint Press

Disclaimer

The information contained in this book is provided for educational and informational purposes only. It is not intended as medical, legal, or professional advice. The author and publisher make no representations or warranties regarding the accuracy, completeness, or applicability of the information and shall not be held liable for any loss, injury, or damage resulting from its use. *This book examines publicly available data, scientific studies, and documented environmental conditions to explore potential connections between environment and public health. It does not allege illegal conduct by any individual or entity, nor does it provide medical or legal advice.*

ISBN: 978-1-969278-03-7
First Edition

Printed in the United States of America

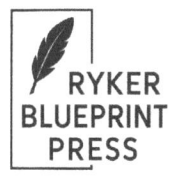

Contents

Dedication	1
Introduction	2
1. A Valley at a Breaking Point	4
2. From River to Faucet	10
3. What's in the Water?	17
4. Toxic Legacy	24
5. The Arroyo Colorado	32
6. Flooding, Drainage, and Failing Infrastructure	39
7. The Air We Breathe	45
8. Public Health in the Valley	51
9. The Future of the Rio Grande Valley	58
10. What Can Be Done	64
11. Conclusion	71
Sources & Notes	77

For my mother, Alma Moroles—

whose resilience continues to inspire me.

Introduction

The Rio Grande Valley has been my home since birth.

Everyone I know and love is here. My family, my friends, the people I've grown up with, the people I work with, and the people I do business with. Every major memory of my life is tied to this place—its streets, its schools, its neighborhoods, its culture. The Valley is not just where I live. It is who I am.

And yet, for as long as I can remember, one question has never left me:

Why are there so many sick people here?

It's a question that doesn't come from statistics or studies—it comes from lived experience. From conversations. From hospital visits. From hearing the same diagnoses repeated across families, neighborhoods, and generations. Cancer. Respiratory illness. Autoimmune disorders. Chronic disease that feels far too common to ignore.

For years, I wondered if it was coincidence. If it was genetics. If it was lifestyle. If it was simply bad luck.

But the more I paid attention, the harder it became to accept that explanation.

This book exists because that question refused to go away.

What you are about to read is not an attack on the Rio Grande Valley. It is an act of care. It is an attempt to step back and look at the region from above—to connect dots that are often discussed separately, if they are discussed at all. Water. Air. Flooding. Infrastructure. Growth. Health.

This book does not claim to have every answer. It is not meant to be the final word. It is one piece of a much larger puzzle.

What it offers is perspective.

An overhead look at some of the biggest challenges facing the Rio Grande Valley—how they overlap, how they compound, and how they quietly shape the health and well-being of the people who live here. Many of these issues have existed for decades. Others are accelerating rapidly. Most have been addressed in fragments, never as a whole.

That fragmentation is part of the problem.

My hope is that this book helps shift the conversation. Away from isolated explanations and toward systemic understanding. Away from silence and toward informed action. Away from the idea that these outcomes are inevitable, and toward the belief that they are not.

I wrote this because I care about this place. Because this is where my life is rooted. And because asking hard questions is sometimes the most honest way to show love for a community.

The Rio Grande Valley deserves clarity.

It deserves accountability.

And it deserves a future where the next generation does not grow up asking the same question I have been asking for years.

This book is my contribution to that effort.

1

A VALLEY AT A BREAKING POINT

For decades, the Rio Grande Valley was known for one thing above all else: agriculture.

Long before sprawling subdivisions, industrial parks, and international trade corridors defined the region, the Valley was farmland—vast, flat, and fertile. By the early 1900s, irrigation projects tied to the Rio Grande transformed South Texas into one of the most productive agricultural regions in the country. Cotton, citrus, sugarcane, sorghum, onions, melons, and vegetables thrived in soil enriched by river sediment and nourished by a subtropical climate.

This productivity didn't happen by accident. It was engineered. Canals were carved, drains were built, and water was diverted to serve crops first. Agriculture fueled economic growth, attracted workers, and anchored communities. Towns grew around packing sheds, rail lines, and irrigation districts. The Valley fed the nation—and in many ways, it fed itself.

But this success came with a cost that would not reveal itself for generations.

Beginning in the mid-20th century—especially between the 1940s and 1970s—industrial-scale farming brought with it heavy pesticide use. Chemicals such as DDT, atrazine, chlordane, and other compounds now known to be toxic or carcinogenic were applied liberally to fields across the region. At the time, these substances were considered modern miracles. They increased yields, controlled pests, and protected profits.

What wasn't understood—or wasn't acknowledged—was what happened after those chemicals were sprayed.

They didn't disappear.

They settled into the soil. They bonded with sediment. They seeped into shallow groundwater. They collected in drainage canals. Even after many of these chemicals were banned nationally in the 1970s and 1980s, their legacy remained embedded in the land itself. The Rio Grande Valley became, quietly and invisibly, a storage site for decades of chemical decisions.

As the years passed, the Valley changed.

Population growth accelerated dramatically in the late 20th and early 21st centuries. From a largely rural region, the Rio Grande Valley evolved into one of the fastest-growing areas in Texas. Cities expanded outward. Colonias emerged on the edges of municipal boundaries. Concrete replaced cropland. Roads, parking lots, and rooftops reshaped how water moved across the land.

But infrastructure did not keep pace.

Drainage systems designed decades earlier for agricultural runoff were suddenly responsible for urban stormwater. Septic systems remained in place as neighborhoods grew denser. Flood control measures lagged behind development. Municipal planning struggled to catch up with the reality on the ground.

And then the floods came—again and again.

The Rio Grande Valley floods often. But to understand why, you must understand one critical truth that is frequently overlooked: the Rio Grande Valley is not a valley at all.

It is a delta.

A delta is a flat, low-lying land form created by sediment deposited over time by a river as it slows and spreads before reaching a larger body of water. Deltas are fertile—but they are also prone to flooding. Water moves slowly. It pools. It lingers. There is little natural elevation to guide it away.

In a true valley, water drains downhill. In a delta, it spreads outward.

This distinction matters because when water floods a delta, it doesn't simply pass through—it interacts with everything in its path.

In the Rio Grande Valley, floodwater doesn't just bring rain. It reactivates the past.

A University of Texas Rio Grande Valley graduate study titled *"Characterization of the Lower Rio Grande Valley Watershed" (May 2023)* connects dots that many residents have lived with for years but never saw fully mapped. The study shows that flooding, drainage, and water contamination are not isolated issues. They stack on top of each other.[1]

When heavy rain falls, water moves through fields, neighborhoods, drainage canals, and flood-ways—picking up what lies dormant in soil and sediment. Pesticides applied decades ago. Industrial chemicals from legacy sites. Runoff from agriculture, roadways, and aging infrastructure.

Flooding doesn't create contamination. It redistributes it.

Water carries these substances into homes, businesses, playgrounds, and schools. It spreads contaminants laterally across communities that

---

1. Findings connecting flooding, elevated bacteria levels, and impaired downstream waters, including the Lower Laguna Madre, from the UTRGV thesis *Characterization of the Lower Rio Grande Valley Watershed*https://scholarworks.utrgv.edu/etd/1190/

may have never directly contributed to their presence. And because floodwaters often sit for days—or weeks—in low-lying areas, exposure is prolonged.

This is not hypothetical. This is how deltas behave.

Yet for years, the narrative has treated flooding, water quality, and public health as separate conversations. Flooding is framed as an inconvenience. Water quality as a technical issue. Health outcomes as personal or genetic misfortune.

The reality is far more interconnected—and far more troubling.

As the Valley grew, the environmental load increased. More people meant more wastewater. More vehicles meant more emissions. More development meant more impervious surfaces that accelerated runoff. At the same time, aging infrastructure strained under demands it was never designed to meet.

Water sat longer. Air stagnated. Contaminants accumulated.

And people got sick.

This is where my personal journey intersects with the Valley's story.

For years, I asked myself a question that many residents quietly ask but rarely say out loud: *Why are there so many sick people in the Rio Grande Valley?*

Cancer. Autoimmune disorders. Asthma. Respiratory illness. Developmental issues in children. Chronic conditions that seem to appear with alarming frequency. Families with multiple diagnoses. Neighborhoods where illness feels normalized—not because it should be, but because it has become common.

I didn't accept that this was coincidence.

I didn't accept that it was simply genetics.

And I didn't accept that a region of over a million people could experience this level of illness without environmental influence.

This book exists because I needed answers—and because too many people have been told to stop asking the question.

As I began to look deeper, a pattern emerged. Not a single cause, but a convergence. Water contamination layered with air pollution. Flooding events layered with chemical exposure. Infrastructure failures layered with rapid growth. Each issue alone might be survivable. Together, they create a cumulative burden on human health.

Water, air, flooding, and health are not separate systems. They are one system.

What enters the soil eventually enters the water. What evaporates or dries becomes airborne dust. What floods redistributes toxins. What is inhaled, ingested, or absorbed accumulates in the body over time. Exposure is not a moment—it is a condition.

And conditions persist.

This chapter is not about assigning blame to a single industry, agency, or generation. It is about acknowledging reality. The Rio Grande Valley's environmental crisis did not appear overnight. It is the result of decades of decisions made in isolation—without considering cumulative impact.

Agriculture fed the region, but it also introduced chemicals that outlived their usefulness. Growth brought opportunity, but it overwhelmed systems meant for a different era. Flooding exposed weaknesses we failed to address. And health outcomes revealed consequences we were unprepared to face.

The environment remembers everything.

So does the human body.

What the reader should understand from this chapter is simple but uncomfortable: the state of our environment is not accidental, and neither are the outcomes we are seeing today. Years of use, overuse, and neglect have shaped the conditions in which we now live.

A VALLEY AT A BREAKING POINT

If nothing changes, those conditions will not remain static—they will worsen.

Children growing up in the Valley today will inherit the cumulative exposure of the past plus the pressures of the future. Their children will inherit even more—unless intervention occurs.

This book is not meant to inspire fear. It is meant to inspire responsibility.

The Rio Grande Valley is not broken beyond repair—but it is at a breaking point. What happens next depends on whether we are willing to see the full picture, connect the dots, and act before the consequences become irreversible.

This chapter begins that conversation.

The chapters that follow will go deeper—into water systems, municipal tap water, toxic sites, flood dynamics, air quality, and public health. But it all starts here, with the land itself, the choices made upon it, and the truth that we can no longer afford to ignore.

The Valley has always been fertile.

The question now is whether it can remain livable.

2

FROM RIVER TO FAUCET

HOW THE RIO GRANDE VALLEY GETS ITS WATER

Water is the one thing no one in the Rio Grande Valley can escape.

We cook with it. We bathe in it. We brush our teeth with it. We wash our clothes, our dishes, our homes, and our children with it. Water is not optional. It is not a luxury. It is life itself.

And for the Rio Grande Valley, nearly all of that life begins in one place: the Rio Grande River.

Stretching more than 1,800 miles from the mountains of Colorado to the Gulf of Mexico, the Rio Grande is not just a geographic boundary between two nations—it is a working river. It is diverted, dammed, pumped, treated, and distributed to serve millions of people on both sides of the border. In the Valley, it is the primary source of municipal drinking water for cities large and small.

Every glass of tap water in the Rio Grande Valley begins its journey there.

What most residents never see—and what few are encouraged to think about—is what that river carries with it before it reaches a treatment plant intake.

The Rio Grande holds a darker secret than many care to realize.

For decades, pollution along the river has been discussed in fragments: agricultural runoff here, industrial discharge there, wastewater issues somewhere upstream. These conversations are often siloed, technical, and abstract. But recent reporting has forced those fragments into a single, uncomfortable picture.

In December 2025, an investigative report titled *"The Big Bet to Fix the Rio Grande Sewage Problem"* documented what communities along the river have long suspected but rarely seen so clearly confirmed: raw and partially treated sewage has been flowing into the Rio Grande in enormous volumes.

According to the report, in Nuevo Laredo, Mexico alone, more than **12 million gallons of raw sewage per day** were leaking into the river prior to wastewater plant repairs. That sewage did not vanish. It flowed downstream. [1]

Water-quality samples collected by the International Boundary and Water Commission revealed **E. coli concentrations as high as 240,000 per 100 milliliters**—nearly **2,000 times higher than Texas' safety standard of 126 per 100 milliliters** for contact recreation.

To put that number into perspective: these are not marginal exceedances. They are orders of magnitude beyond what regulators consider safe even for swimming, much less for a source of drinking water.

The report explicitly states that stretches of the river downstream of wastewater discharges are **unsafe for swimming and contact recreation** due to bacterial contamination. It further documents similar

---

1. Investigative reporting documenting millions of gallons of untreated sewage discharged into the Rio Grande from Nuevo Laredo, published by *Inside Climate News*, July 12, 2025 https://insideclimatenews.org/news/07122025/rio-grande-sewage-pollution-texas-mexico/

sewage-related problems in other urban border regions, including El Paso/Ciudad Juárez, Del Rio/Acuña, Eagle Pass/Piedras Negras, and downstream areas affecting Hidalgo County.

This is not speculation. This is documented journalism grounded in sampling data and agency reports.

And this water keeps moving.

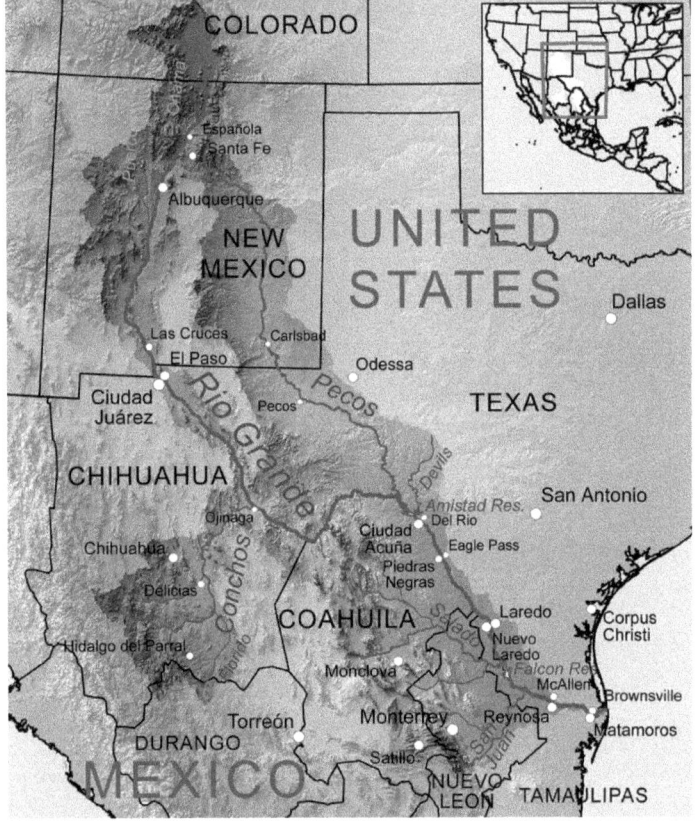

Map from americanrivers.org

By the time the Rio Grande reaches the Valley, it has already absorbed the cumulative impacts of upstream cities, industries, agriculture, and infrastructure failures. It carries bacteria, nutrients, organic waste, industrial chemicals, and sediment—some visible, most not.

This is the water that municipalities withdraw, treat, and send to homes across the region.

Understanding how that happens is critical.

Municipal water systems in the Rio Grande Valley rely on river intakes, reservoirs, and treatment plants designed to remove contaminants and disinfect water before it reaches the tap. In theory, this system works. In practice, it is increasingly strained.

Water is diverted from the river into canals and reservoirs, where it is stored before treatment. At treatment plants, physical processes remove sediment, chemical processes neutralize contaminants, and disinfectants are added to kill bacteria and pathogens.

This process is meant to protect public health.

But it was never designed to handle the scale and complexity of contamination the river now carries.

Many municipalities across the Valley operate **aging treatment facilities**, some built decades ago for much smaller populations and far cleaner source water. As cities expanded rapidly, infrastructure investments often lagged behind growth. Plants were pushed beyond their original design capacity. Pipes aged. Systems became vulnerable.

Flooding makes this worse.

As discussed in Chapter 1, the Rio Grande Valley's delta geography causes water to pool and linger. When heavy rain falls, drainage systems are overwhelmed. Floodwaters infiltrate infrastructure, compromise treatment processes, and increase the load of contaminants entering source water.

During flood events, water systems are not just managing river water—they are managing everything floodwater has touched.

This includes runoff from fields treated with legacy pesticides, industrial sites, roadways, septic systems, and urban surfaces. When treatment plants are overburdened, operators must make difficult choices under pressure: increase chemical dosing, adjust processes, or issue advisories.

In many cases, the solution has been to **over-process the water**—adding more disinfectants and treatment chemicals to ensure the final product meets legal standards.

This is where an uncomfortable truth emerges.

The Rio Grande Valley's water is often so compromised at the source that it must be aggressively treated simply to pass regulatory requirements. This does not necessarily mean it is clean. It means it is compliant.

Compliance is not the same as safety.

Water regulations are based on thresholds, not cumulative exposure. They evaluate individual contaminants in isolation, not the combined effects of dozens of substances interacting over time. They assume average consumption patterns and ideal system performance—conditions that do not always reflect real life.

When treatment plants increase chemical dosing to kill bacteria like E. coli, they trigger chemical reactions with organic matter in the water. These reactions form disinfection byproducts—compounds that are regulated, but only to a point.

This is not a failure of operators. It is a limitation of the system itself.

Many treatment plants in the Valley are doing everything they can with what they have. But they are fighting an upstream problem with downstream tools. No amount of treatment can fully erase what enters the river before it reaches the intake.

And when infrastructure is old, overburdened, or compromised by flooding, the margin for error shrinks.

This is why residents sometimes notice changes in taste, odor, or color in their tap water after storms. This is why boil water notices appear after system disruptions. This is why confidence in the water supply quietly erodes—even when official reports say everything is within limits.

"Treated" does not always mean "safe" in the way people assume it does.

It means the water meets minimum legal thresholds at the point of testing. It does not mean the system upstream is healthy. It does not mean long-term exposure carries no risk. And it does not mean vulnerable populations—children, pregnant women, the elderly—are equally protected.

This chapter is not meant to suggest that tap water in the Rio Grande Valley is instantly toxic or unsafe to drink. It is meant to clarify something more subtle and more important: the system is under strain, and the river it depends on is far more polluted than most residents realize.

The Valley's water story begins long before the faucet is turned on.

It begins upstream, with sewage infrastructure failures, agricultural runoff, industrial discharges, and a river that serves too many needs with too little protection. It continues through treatment plants that must work harder each year to compensate for what they receive. And it ends in homes where people trust that "treated" means harmless.

That trust deserves honesty.

Because the next question is unavoidable: **What remains in the water after treatment?**

What chemicals persist? What byproducts form? How do standards compare to real-world exposure? And how do different municipalities, with different resources and infrastructure, produce very different outcomes?

Those questions lead directly into the next chapter.

This chapter establishes the journey—from river to faucet. The next will examine what survives that journey and enters our bodies every single day.

Because understanding the source is only the beginning.

Understanding what's in the water is where accountability truly begins.

3

WHAT'S IN THE WATER?

TAP WATER QUALITY ACROSS MUNICIPALITIES

Most residents of the Rio Grande Valley learn about their drinking water long after they've already consumed it.

Once a year—usually in the summer—cities release a document called a **Consumer Confidence Report**, or CCR. This report is intended to inform the public about the quality of their tap water. Some municipalities mail it directly to residents. Others post it online, assuming that those who care enough will search for it.

For many people, it arrives quietly in the mail. For others, it never arrives at all.

And even when it does, the most important detail is rarely emphasized: **the report does not reflect current water quality**.

A Consumer Confidence Report summarizes what was detected in the water during the *previous calendar year*. This means that when a resident receives a CCR in the summer of 2026, it documents water conditions from **January 1 through December 31 of 2025**.

That delay is not trivial.

If drinking water was compromised in January—due to flooding, infrastructure failure, source contamination, or treatment disruptions—the public would not learn about it until more than a year later.

By then, the exposure has already occurred. Families have cooked with the water. Children have bathed in it. Infants may have consumed it daily.

This reporting system belongs to a different era—one without real-time monitoring, instant communication, or the environmental pressures the Rio Grande Valley now faces.

Yet it remains the primary mechanism for public disclosure.

Inside every CCR is language that sounds technical, neutral, and reassuring. It explains where drinking water comes from and what it can contain. Nearly identical wording appears year after year:

"The sources of drinking water (both tap and bottled water) include rivers, lakes, streams, ponds, reservoirs, springs, and wells. As water travels over the surface of the land or through the ground, it dissolves naturally occurring minerals and, in some cases, radioactive material, and can pick up substances resulting from the presence of animals or from human activity.

This paragraph appears harmless, even educational. But it quietly acknowledges something most residents are never explicitly told: **drinking water is not pristine when it enters the treatment system**. It is already carrying the cumulative footprint of everything upstream—human, industrial, agricultural, and environmental.

The CCR then lists the categories of contaminants that may be present in source water:

- **Microbial contaminants**, such as viruses and bacteria, often originating from sewage treatment plants, septic systems, agricultural livestock operations, and wildlife.

- **Inorganic contaminants**, including salts and metals, which may occur naturally or result from urban stormwater runoff, industrial or domestic wastewater discharges, oil and gas production, mining, or farming.

- **Pesticides and herbicides**, stemming from agricultural activity, urban runoff, and residential use.

- **Organic chemical contaminants**, including synthetic and volatile organic compounds, which are byproducts of industrial processes and petroleum production, and may also come from gas stations, stormwater runoff, and septic systems.

- **Radioactive contaminants**, which can be naturally occurring or associated with oil, gas, and mining activities.

In other words, the CCR itself confirms what many residents intuitively suspect: **drinking water is vulnerable to contamination long before it is treated**.

For cities like McAllen, the report states plainly that the source of drinking water is **surface water**, supplied by the Falcon and Amistad Dams. Those reservoirs collect Rio Grande water after it has traveled hundreds of miles downstream—through agricultural zones, industrial corridors, border cities, and wastewater discharge points.

This is the starting point for every tap in the Valley.

Some CCRs go even further, including a notice that is often overlooked but deeply significant:

"You may be more vulnerable than the general population to certain microbial contaminants, such as Cryptosporidium, in drinking water. Infants, some elderly, or immunocompromised persons... can be particularly at risk from infections. You should seek advice about drinking water from your physician or health care provider."

This is not a disclaimer for a hypothetical risk. It is an acknowledgment that **certain populations face greater danger from contaminants that may be present even when water meets regulatory standards**.

Understanding what the water is tested for—and how violations occur—requires a closer look at how drinking water is treated.

To kill bacteria and pathogens, municipalities disinfect water using **chlorine or chloramine**. These chemicals are effective and widely used across the United States. Without them, waterborne disease outbreaks would be far more common.

But disinfection comes with tradeoffs.

When chlorine reacts with organic matter already present in the water—material originating from sewage, decaying vegetation, agricultural runoff, or industrial waste—it forms **disinfection byproducts**, commonly referred to as DBPs. These include compounds such as **trihalomethanes (TTHMs)** and **haloacetic acids (HAA5)**. [1]

These byproducts are regulated, but only within defined limits. Over decades, scientific research has consistently shown that **long-term exposure to chlorinated drinking water is associated with increased health risks**, particularly bladder cancer.

This does not mean that one glass of water causes illness. It means that **chronic, low-level exposure over years or decades carries measurable risk**, especially in populations already burdened by environmental stressors.

---

1. Research showing that drinking water disinfection byproducts are associated with additive toxicity and potential health risks, from *Disinfection Byproducts in Drinking Water from the Tap: Variability in Household Calculated Additive Toxicity (CAT)* https://pmc.ncbi.nlm.nih.gov/articles/PMC11320572/

In regions like the Rio Grande Valley—where source water is heavily impacted and treatment plants must work harder to disinfect—DBP formation becomes more likely. The more organic material in the source water, the more byproducts form during disinfection.

This creates a paradox: the dirtier the source water, the more aggressively it must be treated—and the greater the potential for byproducts that carry their own health concerns.

This is not a failure of treatment plant operators. It is a limitation of the system itself.

Beyond disinfection byproducts, CCRs document a range of contaminants that vary by municipality, source conditions, and infrastructure age. These include **arsenic**, **chromium-6**, **nitrates**, **total dissolved solids**, and other inorganic compounds.

Some occur naturally in regional geology. Others are influenced by human activity. What matters is not just their presence, but their **persistence**.

More recently, CCRs across the country—including those in Texas—have begun listing **PFAS**, often referred to as "forever chemicals." These compounds are not new to the environment. They have been used for decades in industrial processes, firefighting foams, nonstick coatings, and consumer products.

What *is* new is the requirement to test for them.

PFAS are now appearing in CCRs not because they suddenly entered the Rio Grande Valley, but because municipalities are finally being required to measure and disclose them. Their detection raises a critical point: **absence from a report does not mean absence from the water**. It often means the contaminant was not tested for.

This creates significant variation across municipalities.

Some cities test more frequently. Some test for a broader list of contaminants. Others meet only the minimum requirements. CCRs may differ not because water quality is dramatically better or worse, but because **reporting practices and system capacity vary**.

This leads to reporting gaps that are difficult for residents to interpret. Two neighboring cities may publish very different-looking reports, even though they draw from the same river.

Regulatory limits further complicate the picture.

Drinking water standards are largely developed by evaluating individual contaminants one at a time. In most cases, these standards do not consider cumulative exposure, interactions between multiple chemicals, or the long-term ingestion of complex mixtures. As a result, water can meet all regulatory requirements while still containing several contaminants at levels just below their individual limits..

Compliance does not equal absence.

It means the system passed a snapshot test at a specific moment in time.

For residents, this distinction is rarely explained. CCRs often emphasize phrases like "meets all state and federal requirements," without clarifying what those requirements do—and do not—protect against.

What residents are being told is that the water is legal.

What they are not being told is how much uncertainty exists within those legal boundaries.

They are not told how often water quality fluctuates after storms. They are not told how infrastructure stress impacts treatment performance. They are not told that some contaminants accumulate in the body over time. And they are not told that many standards are based on decades-old science that is still evolving.

The CCR fulfills a legal obligation, but it does not fully inform the public.

This chapter is not about panic. It is about clarity.

Understanding what's in the water requires more than reading a report once a year. It requires understanding how data is delayed, how contaminants are tested, how treatment alters water chemistry, and how regulations define "safe."

The Rio Grande Valley's water story is not one of instant danger—it is one of **chronic exposure, systemic strain, and incomplete transparency**.

And that leads directly to the next chapter.

Because once we understand what's reported in the water, we must confront what lies beyond reporting—**toxic legacy sites**, contamination that predates modern regulation, and pollutants that move silently through groundwater and soil.

The water does not exist in isolation.

Neither does the risk.

4

TOXIC LEGACY

THE MCALLEN GROUNDWATER PLUME AND SUPERFUND SITES IN THE RIO GRANDE VALLEY

When people hear the term *Superfund site*, they often imagine a distant industrial wasteland—somewhere far removed from daily life. Rusted fences. Warning signs. Places no one visits.

That image does not fit the Rio Grande Valley.

Here, some of the most significant contamination sites sit beneath active roadways, commercial corridors, canals, reservoirs, and neighborhoods. People drive over them every day. Families shop nearby. Children attend school within their reach. And most residents have no idea what lies below.

A Superfund site is a location designated for cleanup because hazardous substances have contaminated soil, groundwater, or surface water to levels that pose a risk to human health or the environment. These sites are not created overnight. They are the result of **years—or decades—of industrial activity, chemical storage, disposal practices, and regulatory blind spots**.

What makes the Rio Grande Valley unique is not just that these sites exist, but that **their effects linger quietly beneath a rapidly growing region**. [1]

The most striking example is the **McAllen Groundwater Plume Not a superfund site**

Most people drive along 23rd Street and Business 83 every day—shopping, working, thriving—without realizing that what lies beneath the pavement is still being actively monitored more than three decades after contamination was first discovered.

The plume was identified in **1990**, originating from leaking underground petroleum storage tanks. Over time, petroleum products migrated through soil and groundwater, creating a subsurface plume of contamination. Since **2009**, the site has been managed under the Texas Commission on Environmental Quality's Petroleum Storage Tank State Lead Program.

Residents are often told that the contamination is "stable and declining."

That phrase sounds comforting.

It is also incomplete.

As of **2026**, the plume is **not gone**.

Recent monitoring data—much of it from **2025**—shows ongoing contamination across a large network of wells. When the numbers are examined closely, the picture changes from reassurance to concern.

Across approximately **80 monitoring wells**:

- **22 wells** still show lab-detected petroleum chemicals, including BTEX and MTBE.

---

1. Groundwater contamination, Superfund sites, and watershed impairment information in the Rio Grande Valley, based on records from the Texas Commission on Environmental Quality (TCEQ) (https://www.tceq.texas.gov/).

- **16 wells** exceed Category 1 cleanup targets, the most protective thresholds tied to potential human exposure.

- **36 wells** show active contamination indicators—either chemical detections or documented presence of free product.

Free product matters.

In **17 wells**, investigators documented **LNAPL**—light non-aqueous phase liquid—meaning **raw petroleum** still exists underground. In **14 of those wells**, sampling could not even be completed because petroleum was physically present. The largest recorded thickness reached **3.30 feet**.

This is not residual staining. This is bulk petroleum.

The most alarming data point should stop any reader cold.

In one monitoring well, **benzene** reached **9.94 milligrams per liter**. The regulatory target for benzene in groundwater is **0.005 milligrams per liter**. That measurement represents **nearly 1,988 times the cleanup target**.

Benzene is not an abstract chemical. It is a **known human carcinogen**, linked to leukemia and other blood disorders. In total, **15 wells** exceeded the benzene target.

This contamination exists beneath one of the busiest commercial corridors in the region.

The reason this matters goes beyond one site.

Groundwater plumes do not stay neatly contained. They move slowly, following subsurface geology, gradients, and pathways created by soil composition and human activity. Over time, contaminants can spread laterally, migrate vertically, and interact with other systems.

In a delta region like the Rio Grande Valley, where groundwater is shallow and flooding is frequent, the potential for redistribution increases.

Flooding does not just affect surface water. It alters pressure gradients underground. It can mobilize contaminants trapped in soil. It can accelerate plume movement. And it can bring contaminated groundwater closer to the surface—closer to people.

The McAllen plume is not an isolated case. It is a visible example of a larger pattern.

Across the Rio Grande Valley, multiple **Superfund and hazardous sites** reflect decades of industrial, agricultural, and commercial activity—often occurring before modern environmental safeguards were in place.

In **Hidalgo County**, one of the most significant sites is the **Donna Reservoir and Canal System**.

This system was designed to support irrigation and water management. Over time, it became a collection point for contaminants from multiple sources. Industrial solvents, pesticides, and other hazardous substances accumulated in sediment and soil. Canals that move water also move pollution—especially during high-flow and flood events.

Because the reservoir and canals intersect with agricultural land, drainage systems, and nearby communities, contamination does not remain confined. Sediment can be disturbed. Water can overflow. Pollutants can be redistributed downstream.

The long-term concern is not just environmental—it is human.

Nearby residents rely on groundwater, surface water, and the surrounding environment. Persistent contaminants increase the risk of exposure through water contact, dust inhalation, and indirect pathways such as food grown in contaminated areas.

Also in Hidalgo County is the **Hayes-Sammons Warehouse** site. From **1945 to 1968**, the facility operated as a commercial-grade pesticide storage site, where large quantities of agricultural chemicals were housed in two warehouse buildings located near Miller Avenue and East Eighth Street on property leased from the Union Pacific Railroad.

During its years of operation, releases from stored pesticide materials allowed contaminants to enter surrounding soils. These chemicals did not dissipate quickly; like many industrial pesticides of that era, they persisted in the environment, raising long-term concerns about soil and potential groundwater impacts.

The site was later addressed under the **Texas state Superfund program**, and remediation activities were completed. Based on current regulatory determinations, **no further Superfund environmental response actions are required**, and the site is **pending deletion from the Superfund registry**.

While remediation has reduced risk, the Hayes-Sammons site remains an important example of how legacy industrial practices—particularly those involving pesticide storage—can leave lasting environmental footprints that require decades of monitoring, assessment, and cleanup before regulatory closure is achieved.

The **Muñoz Borrow Pits** represent another pathway of environmental risk rooted in historical land-use decisions. Borrow pits are excavated areas where soil or aggregate has been removed, often leaving low-lying depressions that can collect water and interact directly with surrounding soils.

At the Muñoz site, this risk is not theoretical. In the late **1950s**, the property owner accepted multiple dump truck loads of soil contaminated with **pesticides and arsenic**. That soil was stockpiled on the property and intended for use as fill material. Decades later, in **1982**, a citizen complaint prompted an inspection and investigation into possible pesticide contamination. Soil sampling conducted by state authorities confirmed the presence of contaminants.

Rather than being removed, the contaminated soil—estimated at approximately **2,500 cubic feet**—was later **spread across a large portion of the property** (roughly 100 by 400 feet) in the mid-1980s during site preparation activities. This action dispersed contaminants over a broader area, increasing the potential for interaction with surface water, groundwater, and sediments.

In environments like the Rio Grande Valley, where shallow groundwater and flooding are common, such sites can act as conduits for contaminant movement. Standing water can mobilize legacy pesticides and metals from soil into surrounding areas, increasing exposure risks for wildlife and, potentially, nearby communities over time.

In **Cameron County**, the **Niagara Chemical site** in **Harlingen** illustrates how historical industrial activity can leave long-lasting environmental impacts, even decades after operations end. From **1946 to 1962**, the facility formulated liquid and dry pesticides, with blending and storage activities continuing until **1968**. These operations involved chemicals that, over time, were released into surrounding soil and groundwater.

As a result of those releases, the site became contaminated with **arsenic, lead, and pesticide compounds**, affecting both surface soils and underlying groundwater. The plant ceased operations, and its buildings were demolished in **1970**, leaving only concrete slab foundations. Prior to formal state involvement, **three 10,000-gallon underground storage tanks** were removed from the property.

In **1987**, the Niagara Chemical site was listed on the **Texas state Superfund registry**, and the Texas Commission on Environmental Quality entered into an agreed order with potentially responsible parties to conduct a remedial investigation and feasibility study. Cleanup activities have since been completed, and regulatory authorities have determined that no further Superfund response actions are required.

Today, the Niagara Chemical site stands as a documented example of how legacy pesticide manufacturing—common in the mid-20th century—can require decades of investigation, remediation, and oversight before environmental risks are addressed and regulatory closure is achieved.

Chemicals from such sites do not remain frozen in place. They volatilize into the air, leach into groundwater, bind to sediments, and travel through interconnected systems.

Across these sites, the types of contamination share common themes:

- **Industrial solvents** capable of migrating long distances underground

- **Hydrocarbons** from petroleum products that persist for decades

- **Heavy metals** that do not degrade and can accumulate in biological systems

These substances pose long-term risks not only to drinking water supplies, but also to air quality and soil health. Volatile compounds can off-gas into indoor spaces. Contaminated soil can become airborne dust. Groundwater contamination threatens wells and surface water interactions.

One of the most frustrating realities for affected communities is the **timeline**.

Superfund cleanups often span decades. Not because the danger disappears quickly—but because remediation is complex, expensive, and slow. Sites are investigated, studied, modeled, remediated in phases, and monitored for years. Funding constraints, legal processes, and technical limitations extend timelines further.

"Stable" does not mean "clean."

"Monitored" does not mean "resolved."

"Contained" does not mean "harmless."

For residents, this means living with uncertainty beneath their feet.

These sites matter because they form part of the Valley's environmental baseline. They interact with flooding. They influence groundwater quality. They compound the challenges faced by water treatment systems already struggling with degraded source water.

They also raise uncomfortable questions about transparency and accountability.

How many people know these sites exist?

How many understand what contaminants are present?

How often are communities informed when conditions change?

This chapter is not about fear—it is about awareness.

The Rio Grande Valley's environmental challenges did not begin with modern growth. They are layered upon decades of legacy contamination that continues to shape risk today.

Understanding these toxic legacies is essential before we can talk honestly about solutions.

Because the water, the land, and the air remember what was done to them.

And until those memories are fully addressed, the future of the Valley remains tied to its past.

5

THE ARROYO COLORADO

A POLLUTED LIFELINE

To understand the environmental crisis of the Rio Grande Valley, one must understand the Arroyo Colorado.

At first glance, it appears unremarkable—a slow-moving ribbon of water cutting across the landscape. Many residents pass it daily without a second thought. Some mistake it for a natural river. Others assume it is simply a drainage canal.

It is neither.

The Arroyo Colorado is a man-altered waterway whose history mirrors the Valley's most consequential environmental decisions.

Originally, the Arroyo Colorado was a natural distributary of the Rio Grande, carrying freshwater eastward across the delta toward the Laguna Madre. This connection sustained wetlands, wildlife, and natural flushing of the system. That changed in the **mid-20th century**, when flood-control and irrigation projects fundamentally altered the region's hydrology.

Between **1949 and 1954**, construction of flood-control levees and irrigation infrastructure severed the Arroyo Colorado's direct connection to the Rio Grande. The channel was reshaped, straightened, and isolated to protect agricultural land and expanding communities from flooding.

The unintended consequence was profound.

Once cut off from the river's natural flow, the Arroyo Colorado lost its primary source of freshwater circulation. What remained was a slow-moving, stagnant channel with limited natural flushing—an ideal environment for pollution to accumulate.

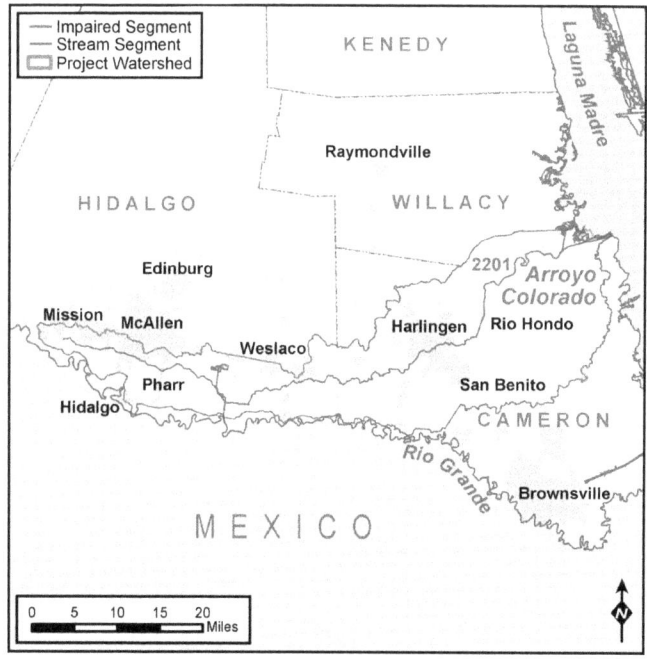

Map from TCEQ Website Arroyo Colorado: Watershed Protection Plan

Over time, the Arroyo Colorado was repurposed.

Today, it functions largely as a **conduit for treated wastewater and stormwater runoff**, carrying effluent eastward until it eventually reaches the **Laguna Madre and the Gulf of Mexico**. This is not speculation. It is documented in state and federal assessments, including the **Arroyo Colorado Watershed Protection Plan**.

Multiple studies by the U.S. Geological Survey and the Texas Commission on Environmental Quality confirm a critical fact: **the Arroyo Colorado's year-round flow is sustained primarily by treated effluent from municipal wastewater treatment facilities**.

In simple terms, the Arroyo flows not because of rainfall or river input, but because cities discharge wastewater into it every single day.

That reality changes how the Arroyo must be understood.

The Arroyo Colorado is officially designated as an **"impaired" water body**. This designation reflects repeated failures to meet water quality standards for its intended uses. Among the documented impairments are **elevated bacteria levels**, **low dissolved oxygen**, and **legacy contaminants** such as **polychlorinated biphenyls (PCBs)** and **mercury**.

These impairments are not isolated incidents. They are structural.

The list of municipalities whose wastewater systems discharge into the Arroyo Colorado watershed reads like a map of the Rio Grande Valley itself: **McAllen, Mission, Pharr, San Juan, Alamo, Donna, Mercedes, Weslaco, La Feria, Harlingen, San Benito, Brownsville, and Rio Hondo**.

Each city operates wastewater treatment facilities designed to remove solids and reduce pathogens before discharge. Under normal conditions, treated effluent meets regulatory requirements. But "treated" does not mean free of contaminants.

Wastewater carries nutrients, bacteria, pharmaceuticals, industrial residues, and chemical byproducts. When released into a **slow-moving, poorly flushed system**, those substances accumulate.

The Arroyo Colorado is not a river that rapidly carries pollution away. It is a channel where contamination lingers.

THE ARROYO COLORADO

Agricultural runoff compounds the problem.

For decades, the surrounding landscape has been shaped by intensive farming. Rainfall washes fertilizers, pesticides, herbicides, and sediments from fields into drainage canals that feed the Arroyo. Even chemicals banned decades ago remain bound to soil and sediments, reentering the water column during storms.

Industrial pollution adds another layer. Facilities near the watershed contribute organic chemicals, metals, and other residues through permitted and accidental releases. Urban stormwater runoff carries oil, heavy metals, tire particles, and debris from roadways and parking lots.

When all of this converges in a single waterway, the result is not dilution—it is concentration.

The Arroyo Colorado's slow flow allows contaminants to settle into sediments. Bacteria thrive. Dissolved oxygen drops, creating conditions hostile to aquatic life. Fish kills have been documented. Wildlife exposure increases. The system becomes a long-term reservoir of pollution.

Flooding makes everything worse.

As discussed in earlier chapters, the Rio Grande Valley's delta geography causes water to spread and linger. During major storms, the Arroyo Colorado overtops its banks. Floodwaters mix with contaminated sediments and spread into nearby neighborhoods, agricultural land, and infrastructure.

Flooding does not introduce new contaminants into the Arroyo. It **redistributes what is already there**.

Power outages and system overloads during major storms further stress wastewater infrastructure. Documented incidents confirm **unauthorized discharges** of partially treated or raw sewage during extreme weather events. These discharges spike bacteria levels and introduce additional organic load into an already burdened system.

The Arroyo Colorado becomes both a recipient and a distributor of pollution.

Recent research has added another disturbing dimension.

In **2024**, scientists identified **PFAS "forever chemicals"** in the Arroyo Colorado. These compounds—used in firefighting foams, industrial processes, and consumer products—do not break down naturally. They persist in water, sediment, and biological tissue.

The highest PFAS concentrations were detected near **potential point sources**, including municipal airports and wastewater treatment facilities. This finding reinforces what the Valley's water story has shown repeatedly: wastewater systems are not designed to remove PFAS, and slow-moving waterways become accumulation zones.

PFAS contamination is especially concerning because of its persistence and its ability to bioaccumulate. Once introduced, it does not leave. It concentrates in fish. It becomes part of the environmental background.

Yet despite all this, the Arroyo Colorado remains one of the most overlooked environmental threats in the Valley.

Why?

Because it does not fit the traditional image of pollution. There are no smokestacks. No warning signs. No dramatic spills that make headlines. Its degradation has been incremental, normalized over decades.

People see water and assume life.

But the Arroyo Colorado's current role is not to sustain ecosystems—it is to manage waste.

That reality has consequences far beyond the banks of the channel.

The Arroyo feeds into the **Laguna Madre**, one of the most ecologically significant hypersaline lagoons in the world. Nutrient loading, bacteria, and chemical contaminants entering this system threaten fisheries, wildlife habitat, and the coastal economy.

The pollution does not stop at the water's edge. Sediments dry and become airborne dust. Volatile compounds off-gas. Floodwaters carry contaminants into homes and schools. The boundary between water quality and public health dissolves.

The Arroyo Colorado illustrates a larger truth about the Rio Grande Valley: **environmental systems do not operate in isolation**.

Agricultural runoff, wastewater discharges, industrial pollution, flooding, air quality, and human health are not separate chapters in a book. They are overlapping layers of the same story.

And yet, the Arroyo remains largely invisible in public discourse.

It is discussed in technical reports, regulatory meetings, and planning documents—but rarely in a way that communicates urgency to the people who live alongside it.

That invisibility is dangerous.

Because the Arroyo Colorado is not just a channel of water. It is a mirror reflecting decades of decisions about growth, infrastructure, and environmental tradeoffs. It shows what happens when a natural system is repurposed without fully accounting for long-term consequences.

This chapter is not about assigning blame to any single city or agency. Every municipality discharging into the Arroyo operates within a system they inherited. But inheritance does not absolve responsibility.

If the Rio Grande Valley is to confront its environmental future honestly, the Arroyo Colorado must be central to the conversation.

It is a lifeline—and it is polluted.

And until that contradiction is addressed, the Valley will continue to live downstream of its own decisions.

6

FLOODING, DRAINAGE, AND FAILING INFRASTRUCTURE

Flooding in the Rio Grande Valley is not an anomaly. It is a recurring condition—and one that has been worsening for years.

When people talk about flooding, it is often framed as a weather problem. Too much rain. A bad storm. An unfortunate event. But in the Rio Grande Valley, flooding is not just about precipitation. It is about infrastructure that has been compromised for decades, systems that were never designed for the growth they now serve, and land-use decisions that ignored hydrology until the consequences became impossible to dismiss.

The floods of **March 2025** made this reality impossible to ignore. Across the Valley, water entered homes, businesses, and schools. Streets became rivers. Drainage systems failed visibly and repeatedly. What was once considered "nuisance flooding" crossed into something far more dangerous: **direct exposure to contaminated floodwater**.

This was not clean rainwater.

Floodwater in the Rio Grande Valley is a complex mixture. It includes stormwater runoff, sewage overflows, agricultural residues, industrial contaminants, petroleum products, and legacy chemicals that have been sitting in soil and sediments for decades. When infrastructure fails, those substances move freely—into living spaces where people assume safety.

One incident in particular crystallized the stakes.

During the March 2025 flooding, water infiltrated an elementary school cafeteria in Edinburg, TX. Floodwater entered food preparation areas—spaces that are supposed to be among the most protected environments for children. Shortly afterward, an **E. coli outbreak** was documented, triggering outrage from parents and the broader community.

The response was swift, emotional, and justified.

But the outbreak itself was not surprising.

It was the predictable result of infrastructure failure meeting contaminated floodwater.

Schools, hospitals, and public buildings across the Valley were never designed to withstand repeated inundation. Many sit in low-lying areas. Many rely on aging drainage connections. When floodwater breaches these spaces, it brings with it whatever contaminants it has encountered upstream.

This is how flooding magnifies pollution exposure.

The Rio Grande Valley's stormwater systems were largely designed for a different era—when cities were smaller, land was more permeable, and rainfall patterns were less extreme. Over time, urbanization has dramatically altered how water moves across the landscape.

As land is developed, natural surfaces that absorb rainfall—soil, vegetation, wetlands—are replaced with concrete, asphalt, and rooftops. These **impervious surfaces** prevent water from soaking into the ground. Instead, rainfall becomes runoff, moving quickly and forcefully into streets, canals, and drainage systems.

The result is higher peak flows, faster flooding, and less margin for error.

This relationship between growth, land use, and flooding has been studied in detail within the Valley itself. Research examining stormwater runoff across multiple cities in the Lower Rio Grande Valley demonstrates that **population growth and land development directly increase runoff volume and flooding risk**.

As urbanization expands, pervious cover decreases. Stormwater systems become overloaded. Retention capacity is exceeded. Overflow moves freely across contaminated surfaces, collecting pollutants along the way.

Floodwater does not discriminate. It travels through neighborhoods, commercial zones, industrial areas, agricultural land, and legacy contamination sites. It mixes with sewage from overwhelmed wastewater systems. It interacts with soil that contains pesticides, hydrocarbons, and heavy metals. And it carries those substances into places people live and work.

Drainage canals—many of which double as floodways—play a central role in this process. Designed to move water away from developed areas, they now serve as conduits for contamination during storms. When these canals overtop, they do not simply spill water. They spill **everything the water has accumulated**.

Retention basins and detention ponds, often promoted as flood-control solutions, are not immune. When improperly sized, poorly maintained, or overwhelmed by extreme rainfall, they fail. Instead of capturing runoff, they become secondary sources of overflow, releasing contaminated water back into the environment.

This is not a hypothetical scenario. It is observable, repeatable, and increasingly common.

Climate change adds another layer of stress.

The Rio Grande Valley is experiencing more frequent **extreme rainfall events**—short-duration storms that deliver large volumes of water in a matter of hours. These events overwhelm systems that were designed for slower, less intense rainfall patterns. When rainfall exceeds design capacity, infrastructure fails by default.

At the same time, prolonged drought periods harden soil and reduce infiltration, making runoff even more severe when rain does arrive. The combination of drought and deluge creates a system that oscillates between extremes, leaving little room for recovery.

Urban growth compounds this instability.

Development has often outpaced planning. New subdivisions, commercial centers, and industrial projects increase runoff without proportionate investment in stormwater infrastructure. Drainage improvements are frequently reactive—implemented after damage occurs rather than before risk materializes.

The result is a patchwork system where some areas receive upgrades while others remain vulnerable. Flooding shifts from one neighborhood to another, creating cycles of damage rather than resolution.

Infrastructure investments lag behind risk for several reasons.

Stormwater systems are largely invisible. Unlike roads or buildings, they are buried underground or hidden in canals. Their failure is only noticed when flooding occurs—and even then, attention often fades once water recedes.

Funding mechanisms are fragmented. Stormwater management competes with other priorities such as road repair, public safety, and economic development. In many cases, cities rely on limited drainage fees or bond funding that falls short of addressing systemic needs.

There is also a political challenge. Investing in drainage does not produce immediate, visible returns. It prevents disasters rather than showcasing progress. That makes it harder to justify large expenditures—until the cost of inaction becomes undeniable.

The March 2025 floods made that cost visible.

Homes were damaged. Businesses closed temporarily or permanently. Schools were disrupted. And exposure risks multiplied across the region.

What made this flooding particularly dangerous was not just the volume of water—it was **what the water carried**.

Floodwater in the Rio Grande Valley often contains elevated bacteria levels due to sewer overflows and wastewater system stress. It can contain petroleum residues from roadways and commercial corridors. It can mobilize pesticides and herbicides from agricultural land. It can disturb contaminated sediments from canals, reservoirs, and legacy sites.

When floodwater enters a home, it does not leave contamination behind when it drains away. Residues remain on surfaces, in carpets, in drywall, and in soil. Mold growth follows. Indoor air quality deteriorates. Health risks persist long after the storm.

For vulnerable populations—children, the elderly, and those with compromised immune systems—the risks are magnified.

The elementary school cafeteria incident is not an isolated case. It is a warning.

It demonstrates how environmental systems intersect with public spaces in ways that are often overlooked until harm occurs. It shows how infrastructure failure can translate directly into health consequences. And it underscores the reality that **flooding is not just an inconvenience—it is a vector for exposure**.

This chapter is not about blaming rainfall or climate alone. It is about recognizing that flooding in the Rio Grande Valley is the result of **human decisions layered onto natural vulnerability**.

The Valley's delta geography means water will always be part of the landscape. But how that water moves, where it accumulates, and what it carries are shaped by infrastructure choices.

For too long, those choices have underestimated risk.

As growth continues, the margin for error shrinks. Without substantial investment in stormwater systems, drainage canals, retention capacity, and coordinated regional planning, flooding will continue to expose communities to contamination.

And as climate pressures intensify, the consequences will escalate.

Flooding is the mechanism that connects water contamination, soil pollution, air quality, and public health. It is the force that mobilizes what has been buried, diluted, or ignored.

If the Rio Grande Valley is to confront its environmental reality honestly, it must stop treating flooding as a temporary crisis and start treating it as a **chronic infrastructure failure**.

Because when the water rises, it carries the Valley's past into its present—and deposits it squarely into its future.

7

THE AIR WE BREATHE

AN INVISIBLE THREAT

There is a statistic that should stop every reader cold.

According to compiled emissions data published by **RGV Health Connect**, **from 2013 through 2024, Cameron County released more than 300,000 pounds of recognized carcinogens into the air**. Over the same period, its neighboring county—sharing the same region, climate, and population pressures—released only a **tiny fraction** of that amount. [1]

Most people in Cameron County do not know this.

Most people in the Rio Grande Valley do not know this.

And yet, this data exists—quietly compiled, publicly available, and largely ignored.

Air pollution has a way of hiding in plain sight. Unlike contaminated water, which can discolor, smell, or taste different, polluted air often looks normal. You breathe it without thinking. You inhale it without permission. And over time, it becomes part of your body.

---

1. Air emissions data showing more than 300,000 pounds of carcinogenic releases in Cameron County from 2013–2024, sourced from RGV Health Connect (https://www.rgvhealthconnect.org/).

The sheer scale of carcinogenic emissions in Cameron County is not the result of a single event. It is the cumulative effect of **industrial activity, energy production, transportation, agriculture, and regulatory decisions** layered year after year.

Air pollution does not remain confined to fence lines or city limits. It moves with wind patterns. It settles on soil and water. It enters homes through doors, windows, and ventilation systems. And it does so continuously.

Cameron County sits at the intersection of several major air quality stressors—some visible, many not.

One of the most disruptive forces reshaping the region is the rapid expansion of **industrial and energy infrastructure** along the coast. Brownsville, Texas, has become the focal point for major liquefied natural gas projects. These developments are transforming the Port of Brownsville into a global energy export hub.

Large-scale LNG facilities are not quiet neighbors.

They bring increased ship traffic, flaring, combustion processes, and continuous emissions of pollutants associated with natural gas processing. Volatile organic compounds, nitrogen oxides, particulate matter, and hazardous air pollutants become part of the background atmosphere.

These projects are often framed in economic terms—jobs, investment, growth. What receives far less attention is the **long-term air quality burden** placed on nearby communities.

Once built, these facilities operate around the clock. Emissions are not episodic. They are persistent.

The impacts extend beyond the immediate industrial zone. South Padre Island, long celebrated for its beaches, wildlife, and tourism, exists downwind of this transformation. Changes in air quality, haze, odors, and deposition do not stop at the port.

The South Padre Island of the future will not be the same as the one people remember—because air pollution does not respect nostalgia.

Another major contributor to air quality degradation in Cameron County comes from **aerospace and rocket activity**. Launch operations, testing, and associated industrial processes release a complex mix of combustion byproducts and particulate matter.

Rocket launches are dramatic and brief, but their environmental footprint does not end when the sound fades. Combustion products can disperse widely, settle into surrounding ecosystems, and contribute to cumulative exposure over time.

Add to this the emissions from **power plants**, industrial boilers, diesel engines, and heavy truck traffic supporting these industries, and the air becomes a layered mixture of pollutants.

Agriculture contributes its own share.

Burning of agricultural waste, application of chemicals, and dust from tilled fields release particulate matter into the atmosphere. These particles are small enough to remain suspended and inhaled deep into the lungs.

The Rio Grande Valley's geography amplifies these effects. Flat terrain and temperature inversions can trap pollutants near the ground, especially during calm weather conditions. What rises does not always disperse.

Cross-border pollution adds another dimension.

The Rio Grande Valley is not isolated. It shares air with **Matamoros and Reynosa**, two densely populated border cities with their own industrial, commercial, and residential emissions. Open burning, waste fires, industrial activity, and vehicular emissions across the border do not stop at the river.

Particles and toxic fumes cross freely into the Valley, carried by prevailing winds. On some days, residents can smell smoke or chemical odors without any visible local source. The pollution is real, but its origin is harder to pinpoint—and therefore easier to dismiss.

Air pollution does not carry a passport.

One of the most dangerous components of air pollution is **fine particulate matter**, known as **PM2.5**. These particles are smaller than 2.5 micrometers—small enough to bypass the body's natural defenses and lodge deep in the lungs or enter the bloodstream.

PM2.5 comes from combustion: vehicle exhaust, industrial processes, power generation, agricultural burning, and wildfires. It is associated with increased risk of heart disease, stroke, asthma, and premature death.

Ozone is another major concern.

Ground-level ozone forms when emissions from vehicles and industrial sources react in sunlight. It is not emitted directly, which makes it harder for the public to understand. Ozone irritates the respiratory system, reduces lung function, and exacerbates asthma and other chronic conditions.

Volatile organic compounds—VOCs—play a central role in both ozone formation and direct toxicity. Many VOCs are carcinogenic. Others cause neurological, respiratory, and developmental effects. They are emitted by refineries, chemical plants, fuel storage, solvents, and industrial operations.

In Cameron County, these pollutants do not exist in isolation. They exist together.

The health implications are profound.

Air pollution has been linked to **asthma, chronic obstructive pulmonary disease, cardiovascular disease, cancer, low birth weight, and developmental issues in children**. These are not rare conditions in the Rio Grande Valley. They are familiar diagnoses.

And yet, air quality often receives less attention than water.

There are several reasons for this.

Water quality is tangible. You can test it. You can bottle it. You can see advisories and boil notices. Air pollution is invisible. Its effects accumulate silently over years.

Air quality monitoring stations are fewer and farther between. Data is averaged over time. Short-term spikes can be smoothed out, making conditions appear better than they feel.

There is also a psychological barrier. People assume air pollution is a problem for big cities, not coastal communities or rural regions. The Valley does not look like an industrial skyline—so the threat is underestimated.

But the numbers tell a different story.

Releasing **hundreds of thousands of pounds of carcinogens into the air** over a decade is not incidental. It is structural.

It reflects policy decisions about where heavy industry is placed, how emissions are regulated, and whose health is prioritized. It reflects a willingness to accept environmental burden in exchange for economic development—often without fully accounting for cumulative impact.

Air pollution compounds every other environmental stress discussed in this book.

Particles settle into water bodies. They deposit onto soil. They enter floodwaters. They are inhaled during storms when people clean up damage. They exacerbate health vulnerabilities already shaped by water contamination and flooding exposure.

This is why air quality cannot be treated as a separate issue.

It is part of the same system.

The Rio Grande Valley's environmental challenges are converging. Water contamination, failing infrastructure, flooding, toxic legacy sites, and air pollution are not isolated chapters. They reinforce one another.

Ignoring air quality because it is invisible does not make it less dangerous.

If anything, it makes it easier to normalize.

This chapter is not about predicting catastrophe. It is about recognizing patterns.

When carcinogenic emissions accumulate year after year…

When industrial development accelerates faster than environmental oversight…

When communities downwind are told exposure is acceptable because it is legal…

The outcome is not uncertainty. It is a predictable trajectory.

Air pollution does not announce itself. It does not knock. It enters quietly, breath by breath.

And in Cameron County—and across the Rio Grande Valley—it has been doing so for a very long time.

This book does not allege illegal activity, but examines cumulative environmental impact within existing regulatory frameworks.

8

PUBLIC HEALTH IN THE VALLEY

THE HUMAN COST

If the earlier chapters explain *how* the Rio Grande Valley became environmentally burdened, this chapter confronts the unavoidable question of *what that burden has done to the people who live here*.

The answer is not abstract. It is not theoretical. It is measurable in diagnoses, hospital admissions, prescription bottles, missed school days, lost work, and early deaths.

The Rio Grande Valley carries a disproportionate share of illness—and that burden falls heaviest on those with the fewest resources to escape it.

*The conditions discussed in this chapter are not presented as being caused by any single factor. Rather, decades of research show that environmental exposures are **associated with increased risk** for certain diseases, particularly when combined with poverty, limited healthcare access, and long-term cumulative exposure.*

*In the Rio Grande Valley, elevated rates of certain conditions—**including cancers, asthma, respiratory disease, cardiovascular disease, diabetes, and autoimmune disorders**—have been **consistently associated with environmental exposure, socioeconomic stressors, and barriers to preventive care**.*

Across the region, rates of **cancer, respiratory disease, heart disease, diabetes, obesity, and autoimmune disorders** exceed state and national averages in ways that cannot be explained by individual choice alone. These conditions cluster geographically, socially, and generationally.

The pattern points outward—to environment, access, and exposure.

Cancer offers the clearest example.

The Rio Grande Valley has some of the **highest cervical cancer rates in the United States**, particularly in Hidalgo and Starr counties. What makes this especially troubling is not just the incidence, but the **stage at which the disease is diagnosed**. Late-stage diagnoses are common. Mortality rates remain high.

Cervical cancer is one of the most preventable cancers. Screening and early detection save lives. When a region shows persistently high rates of late-stage disease, it signals systemic failure—not personal neglect.

Liver and gallbladder cancers represent another alarming trend. The Valley has a recognized cluster of liver disease, including non-alcoholic fatty liver disease, which can progress to cirrhosis and liver cancer. These conditions are closely tied to metabolic disorders, environmental stressors, and chronic inflammation.

Colorectal cancer is also rising in the region. While it is often described as linked to "modifiable risk factors," that framing ignores the context in which those risks develop. Obesity, diabetes, and physical inactivity do not occur in a vacuum. They are shaped by environment, access to healthy food, safe places to exercise, and consistent healthcare.

Cancer is only one part of the picture.

Asthma and chronic respiratory illness are widespread in the Valley. Emergency room visits for asthma flare-ups are common, particularly among children. These conditions are exacerbated by **air pollution, particulate matter, ozone exposure, mold following flooding, and indoor air contamination**.

For children growing up in the Rio Grande Valley, exposure begins early.

Children breathe more air per pound of body weight than adults. They drink more water relative to their size. Their organs and immune systems are still developing. This makes them especially vulnerable to environmental contaminants.

When floodwater enters homes, when mold grows unchecked, when air quality worsens, children absorb those exposures during critical developmental windows. The consequences may not appear immediately. They may emerge years later as chronic disease.

Autoimmune disorders add another layer of complexity.

While autoimmune diseases are influenced by genetics, environmental triggers play a significant role. Chronic exposure to pollutants—through water, air, and soil—can dysregulate immune function. In regions with multiple overlapping exposures, autoimmune conditions appear more frequently and often more severely.

Heart disease and diabetes are often described as lifestyle-related illnesses. In the Rio Grande Valley, that description is incomplete.

The Valley has some of the **highest rates of diabetes and obesity in Texas**. These conditions are influenced by diet and physical activity—but also by chronic stress, environmental toxins, food deserts, and limited access to preventive care.

Environmental exposure can worsen insulin resistance, promote inflammation, and compound metabolic dysfunction. When combined with poverty and limited healthcare access, these effects become entrenched.

Poverty is not a side note in this story. It is central.

The Rio Grande Valley has some of the **highest poverty rates in the United States**. Family poverty rates hover between **20 and 25 percent**, nearly double—or in some areas triple—the national average. Counties such as Starr, Hidalgo, Willacy, and Cameron routinely rank among the poorest in the nation.

In parts of the Valley, **more than 30 percent of residents live below the federal poverty line**. Child poverty is especially severe, with entire communities where poverty is the norm rather than the exception.

Poverty shapes health in powerful ways.

People living in poverty are more likely to live near contaminated sites, flood-prone areas, and industrial corridors. They are less likely to have health insurance. They are more likely to delay care because of cost, transportation barriers, or fear of medical debt.

Preventive care becomes a luxury.

Screenings are postponed. Symptoms are ignored until they become unbearable. Conditions that could have been managed early progress into crises.

Colonias illustrate this burden starkly.

Colonias—often unincorporated communities lacking basic infrastructure—face compounded environmental and health risks. Many lack adequate drainage, paved roads, or reliable water and sewer systems. Flooding is frequent. Standing water persists. Mold growth is common.

Residents of colonias often rely on septic systems vulnerable to failure during storms. When floodwater mixes with sewage, exposure becomes unavoidable. Children play where water lingers. Families track contamination into homes.

Healthcare access in these areas is limited. Transportation barriers, language barriers, and distrust of systems that have historically failed these communities further delay care.

The result is a cycle of exposure and illness that spans generations.

Healthcare systems in the Valley operate under constant strain.

Hospitals and clinics serve populations with high disease burden and limited resources. Emergency rooms become primary care for many. Chronic conditions require long-term management in a system already stretched thin.

Healthcare providers in the region work tirelessly to address these challenges. Community education programs, mobile clinics, and early detection initiatives exist—and they matter. But they are working upstream against environmental and social forces that continue to generate new cases faster than they can be prevented.

This is not a failure of doctors or nurses. It is a failure of conditions.

Generational health impacts are already visible.

Children raised in environments with persistent pollution and poverty face higher risks of chronic disease as adults. Pregnant women exposed to air and water contaminants face higher risks of complications, low birth weight, and developmental impacts.

These outcomes do not reset with each generation. They accumulate.

When people ask why the Rio Grande Valley seems to carry so much illness, the answer is not singular. It is cumulative.

It is the result of:

- **Long-term environmental exposure**

- **Chronic infrastructure failure**

- **Air and water contamination**

- **Flooding and mold**

- **Poverty and limited access to care**

- **Delayed diagnosis and treatment**

The environment sets the baseline. Social conditions determine who bears the cost.

This chapter is not meant to suggest that every illness in the Valley is caused by environmental exposure. Human health is complex. Genetics matter. Behavior matters. Chance matters.

But to ignore the role of environment in shaping health outcomes in the Rio Grande Valley is to ignore overwhelming evidence.

The Valley is not just facing a public health challenge. It is facing a **public health legacy**—one created over decades and passed quietly from one generation to the next.

If earlier chapters asked *where the contamination is* and *how it moves*, this chapter answers *who it reaches*.

The human cost is not evenly distributed. It is borne disproportionately by children, low-income families, colonias, and communities with the least political power.

This is why environmental justice is not a slogan here. It is a necessity.

The Valley's future health depends not only on better medicine, but on better environments. It depends on addressing water quality, air pollution, flooding, infrastructure, and legacy contamination together—not as separate problems, but as a single system.

Because as long as that system remains unchanged, the human cost will continue to rise.

And the next generation will inherit not just the land—but the consequences of how it was treated.

Understanding these associations does not mean assigning single causes, but recognizing how environment, access, and exposure combine over time to shape population health.

9

THE FUTURE OF THE RIO GRANDE VALLEY

IF NOTHING CHANGES

The Rio Grande Valley is special.

It is culturally rich, biologically unique, binational, and resilient. It has survived droughts, floods, hurricanes, and economic neglect. Families have built lives here for generations, adapting to hardship with creativity and endurance.

But resilience has limits.

Today, the Valley is caught in a mindset that threatens to push those limits beyond recovery: **growth at any cost**.

Across the region—especially in Cameron County—massive projects are being approved and promoted under the banner of economic development, often without a serious accounting of environmental strain. Two enormous data centers are moving forward. Industrial energy hubs are expanding. LNG terminals, power-intensive facilities, and infrastructure-heavy developments are accelerating.

Each project is evaluated individually. Rarely are they assessed cumulatively.

That is the danger.

Data centers alone are among the most **water- and energy-intensive facilities** in modern industry. They require enormous amounts of electricity to operate and vast quantities of water to cool equipment. In a region already facing water stress, aging infrastructure, and rising energy demand, this is not a neutral choice.

It is a bet.

And the Valley is placing that bet without the margin to absorb loss.

One of the most misunderstood realities about water in the Rio Grande Valley is this: **we will not run out of water—we will run out of cheap water**.

That distinction matters.

The Rio Grande has always been a contested and carefully managed resource. Droughts are not new. What is new is the combination of prolonged drought, upstream depletion, population growth, industrial demand, and climate volatility.

As water becomes scarcer and more polluted, treatment costs rise. Infrastructure upgrades become unavoidable. Energy costs for pumping, treating, and distributing water increase. Eventually, those costs are passed on to consumers.

In wealthier regions, rising water bills are an inconvenience.

In the Rio Grande Valley, they are a crisis.

This is a region where poverty rates exceed state and national averages. Where many families already choose between rent, food, healthcare, and utilities. Where water affordability is not theoretical—it is daily math.

Now layer onto that reality an aging water system that must work harder every year to deliver "compliant" water. Add drought-driven scarcity. Add industrial users who can outbid municipalities for supply. Add energy-hungry facilities that strain the grid.

The result is not hypothetical.

It is predictable.

Ten Years From Now

If nothing changes, the Rio Grande Valley in ten years will look familiar—but strained.

Water rates will rise steadily. Not dramatically at first, but persistently. Small increases compounded year after year. For many families, affordability will quietly erode.

Boil water notices will become more frequent after storms. Infrastructure failures will be normalized. Flooding will continue to expose homes, schools, and businesses to contaminated water, especially in low-lying and unincorporated areas.

Health outcomes will worsen subtly but unmistakably.

Asthma rates will continue to climb as air pollution increases and mold exposure follows repeated flooding. Cancer diagnoses will remain high, with late-stage detection still common in underserved communities. Diabetes and heart disease will further burden families already stretched thin.

Healthcare systems will absorb the pressure—for a while.

Emergency rooms will remain crowded. Clinics will operate at capacity. Providers will treat symptoms faster than root causes can be addressed.

Economically, the Valley will appear to be "growing," but the benefits will be uneven. High-energy industries will operate efficiently behind fences. Construction jobs will come and go. Permanent employment gains will be limited.

Meanwhile, workforce health will decline.

Workers dealing with chronic illness, caregiving responsibilities, and untreated conditions will miss more work. Productivity will suffer. Employers will quietly struggle to find and retain healthy labor and possibly move to robotics and artificial intelligence.

Migration will begin towards Hidalgo County —not as a mass exodus, but as a slow bleed.

Families who can afford to leave will do so, seeking regions with better infrastructure, cleaner environments, and lower long-term risk. Those who remain will be those with the fewest options.

Environmental injustice will deepen.

Twenty Years From Now

If nothing changes, the Valley in twenty years will face consequences that are no longer manageable with incremental fixes.

Water will still flow—but at a price many cannot afford.

Advanced treatment technologies, desalination, and infrastructure overhauls will be unavoidable. These solutions are expensive. They require enormous energy input. They demand long-term investment.

Without proactive planning, the cost burden will fall disproportionately on residents least able to pay.

Some communities will face water insecurity—not because water does not exist, but because access becomes financially or logistically constrained.

Flooding will be more severe and more destructive.

Climate patterns suggest fewer moderate rains and more extreme events. Stormwater systems already overwhelmed will fail more often. Contaminated floodwater will continue to enter homes and public buildings. Repeated exposure will make certain neighborhoods effectively uninhabitable without massive intervention.

Health impacts will compound across generations.

Children exposed today will become adults with higher baseline disease risk. Chronic illness will no longer be an exception—it will be the norm. Healthcare costs will soar, consuming household income and public resources.

The Valley's healthcare system will struggle to keep up, not because providers are insufficient, but because the environmental drivers of disease remain unaddressed.

Economically, the Valley will face a reckoning.

Healthcare costs will consume a growing share of household and public budgets. Workforce participation will decline as chronic illness increases. Employers will factor environmental risk into location decisions.

Tourism—especially coastal tourism—will suffer as air quality, water quality, and ecosystem health decline. South Padre Island, long a symbol of natural beauty and escape, will not be immune to industrialization and environmental degradation.

Environmental injustice will become permanent.

Once communities are locked into cycles of contamination, flooding, illness, and poverty, escape becomes nearly impossible without outside intervention. Property values decline. Investment bypasses. Political influence weakens.

The Valley risks becoming a region where environmental burden is no longer debated—only endured.

This Is a Warning, Not Speculation

Nothing in this projection is radical. Nothing relies on worst-case assumptions. Every outcome described here is the logical extension of conditions already documented in this book.

We have already seen:

- Water systems pushed beyond design limits

- Flooding that spreads contamination
- Air pollution measured in hundreds of thousands of pounds of carcinogens
- Persistent health disparities tied to environment and access
- Infrastructure investments lagging behind growth

The future does not arrive suddenly. It accumulates.

The Rio Grande Valley stands at a crossroads.

One path continues the current trajectory: approving projects in isolation, deferring infrastructure investment, externalizing environmental costs, and assuming resilience will carry the load.

The other path requires something more difficult: restraint, coordination, transparency, and long-term planning rooted in environmental reality.

This chapter exists to make one thing clear.

If nothing changes, the Valley's challenges will not plateau. They will intensify. And the people who pay the highest price will be those who have already paid the most.

The question is no longer whether growth will come.

The question is **what kind of future that growth will leave behind**.

Because once the costs are locked in—once infrastructure collapses, ecosystems degrade, and health outcomes harden—there is no shortcut back.

The environment always collects its debt.

And the Rio Grande Valley is approaching a due date.

10

WHAT CAN BE DONE

SOLUTIONS, ACCOUNTABILITY, AND ACTION

The Rio Grande Valley does not suffer from a lack of information.

It suffers from a lack of **action, coordination, and transparency**.

Every problem described in this book—contaminated water, polluted air, flooding, failing infrastructure, and public health disparities—has been documented in some form. Reports exist. Studies exist. Data exists.

What has been missing is a system that connects knowledge to accountability in real time.

This chapter is not about blame. It is about what can be done—now—before the Valley's environmental debt becomes unpayable.

The First Fix: Ending Outdated Water Reporting

One of the most dangerous failures described in this book is the **antiquated Consumer Confidence Report system**.

Residents receive water quality data once a year—often more than twelve months after exposure has already occurred. In a region facing flooding, contamination, and infrastructure stress, this delay is unacceptable.

This is not a technological problem. It is a governance problem.

The tools to fix this already exist.

Blockchain technology offers a direct solution.

Blockchain is not about speculation or finance. At its core, it is a **decentralized, tamper-resistant ledger**. When applied to environmental monitoring, it can record water quality data in real time, permanently, transparently, and without the ability to alter results after the fact.

Imagine a system where:

- Water sampling results are uploaded immediately

- Data is timestamped and immutable

- Residents can view current water quality on demand

- Historical trends are publicly accessible

- Manipulation, delay, or selective reporting is impossible

Instead of waiting a year to learn what was in their water, residents would know **now**.

This would not replace laboratories, treatment plants, or regulation. It would strengthen them by restoring trust and enabling rapid response.

Real-time transparency protects people.

Policy Reforms and Regulatory Improvements

Transparency alone is not enough. Policy must catch up to reality.

Regulatory systems were designed for a time when environmental threats were slower, more localized, and easier to isolate. The Rio Grande Valley now faces **compound risks**—multiple stressors acting at once.

Policy reform must reflect this complexity.

First, cumulative impact must be considered in permitting decisions. Projects should not be approved in isolation. Industrial facilities, data centers, power plants, and infrastructure expansions must be evaluated based on **combined water use, energy demand, emissions, and flood risk**.

Second, water quality standards should move beyond single-contaminant thresholds. Real-world exposure involves mixtures, long-term ingestion, and vulnerable populations. Regulations must reflect chronic exposure—not just acute toxicity.

Third, emergency response requirements must be strengthened. Flooding events, system failures, and unauthorized discharges should trigger immediate public notification—not months or years later.

Finally, environmental justice must be codified, not implied. Communities with high poverty, colonias, and flood-prone areas should receive **greater protection**, not greater burden.

Policy should reduce risk—not redistribute it downward.

Infrastructure Investment Priorities

Infrastructure is where policy meets reality.

The Rio Grande Valley's water, drainage, and wastewater systems are operating beyond their intended lifespan. Patchwork repairs and incremental upgrades are no longer sufficient.

Investment must be strategic.

First priority: **stormwater and drainage systems**. Flooding is the mechanism that mobilizes contamination across the Valley. Improving drainage, expanding retention, and restoring natural absorption areas reduce risk across every other system.

Second priority: **water treatment modernization**. As source water quality declines, treatment plants must work harder. Investments should focus on reducing reliance on chemical overprocessing and increasing resilience during storms and power disruptions.

Third priority: **wastewater infrastructure**. Aging systems contribute directly to waterway contamination and flood exposure. Reducing overflows and unauthorized discharges protects both water quality and public health.

Fourth priority: **energy resilience**. Water systems depend on electricity. As energy demand rises, infrastructure must be protected from outages that compromise treatment and monitoring.

These investments are expensive—but so is inaction.

Every dollar deferred today becomes multiple dollars in healthcare costs, disaster recovery, and lost productivity tomorrow.

Transparency, Monitoring, and Real-Time Data

Transparency must become a design principle, not a public relations exercise.

Real-time monitoring of water quality, air pollution, and flooding conditions should be standard—not experimental.

Data should be:

- Publicly accessible

- Easy to understand

- Updated continuously

- Geographically specific

When residents can see conditions change, they can protect themselves. When policymakers can see trends in real time, they can intervene earlier.

This also restores credibility.

People lose trust when information is delayed, minimized, or buried in technical language. Transparency rebuilds trust not by reassurance, but by honesty.

Blockchain-based reporting, open dashboards, and independent verification are tools—not threats—to good governance.

Community Advocacy and Public Engagement

No solution succeeds without public involvement.

For too long, environmental decisions in the Valley have been made in rooms most residents never enter, using language most residents never hear.

That must change.

Community advocacy does not require everyone to become an expert. It requires systems that welcome participation.

Residents should:

- Attend city and utility meetings
- Ask where water comes from and where waste goes
- Demand cumulative impact assessments
- Request real-time data access
- Support policies that prioritize long-term health

Education matters—but empowerment matters more.

Communities that understand risk can demand protection. Communities kept in the dark absorb harm quietly.

A Roadmap for Leaders, Residents, and Future Generations

This book has documented what happens when environmental systems are ignored, fragmented, or deferred.

This final chapter exists to show that the path forward is not mysterious.

It requires:

- **Modernizing transparency** through real-time data and immutable reporting

- **Reforming policy** to reflect cumulative risk and environmental justice

- **Investing in infrastructure** where it prevents the most harm

- **Engaging communities** as partners, not afterthoughts

- **Planning for future generations**, not just the next project

The Rio Grande Valley does not need to choose between growth and health.

It needs to choose **responsible growth**.

Growth that respects water limits.

Growth that accounts for air quality.

Growth that does not externalize costs onto children and the poor.

Growth that strengthens resilience instead of exploiting it.

The Valley's future is still being written.

But time matters.

Every year of delay hardens outcomes. Every flood redistributes contamination. Every untreated exposure accumulates in bodies that cannot opt out.

The environment does not negotiate.

It responds.

This chapter is not a conclusion. It is an invitation.

To leaders: plan beyond election cycles.

To institutions: prioritize transparency over convenience.

To residents: demand accountability before damage becomes permanent.

To future generations: inherit a Valley that chose to protect itself.

What can be done is no longer the question.

What remains is whether we are willing to do it—together—before the cost of waiting becomes irreversible.

The Rio Grande Valley is still worth saving.

But it will not save itself.

11

CONCLUSION

CHOOSING THE VALLEY'S FUTURE

The Rio Grande Valley is often described as resilient. That word appears again and again—after floods, after storms, after economic hardship, after public health crises. Resilience has become a compliment, a badge of honor, and sometimes a convenient excuse.

But resilience alone is not a plan.

This book has not been about isolated failures or unlucky circumstances. It has been about systems—how they were built, how they were neglected, and how their consequences now overlap in ways that affect nearly every resident of the Valley. Water contamination, air pollution, flooding, failing infrastructure, toxic legacy sites, and public health disparities are not separate problems. They are interconnected outcomes of decades of decisions made without full accountability.

The most important truth to take from this book is also the most empowering one: **this crisis is not inevitable**.

It is solvable.

But only if the Valley chooses to treat it that way.

Reframing the Crisis as a Solvable Problem

For too long, the environmental and health challenges of the Rio Grande Valley have been framed as unfortunate realities—side effects of growth, geography, poverty, or border dynamics. That framing is dangerous because it suggests permanence. It implies that these conditions are simply "how things are here."

They are not.

Every issue outlined in this book has solutions that already exist. Modern water treatment technologies. Smarter stormwater management. Real-time environmental monitoring. Stronger permitting standards. Transparent data systems. Coordinated regional planning. Public health interventions that address root causes rather than symptoms.

The problem has never been a lack of tools.

The problem has been a lack of urgency, coordination, and political will.

Reframing the crisis means rejecting the idea that the Valley must choose between growth and health, or between economic development and environmental protection. Those are false choices. Regions across the country—and across the world—have demonstrated that responsible growth is not only possible, but more sustainable in the long term.

It also means acknowledging that incremental fixes are no longer enough. Patchwork repairs, delayed reporting, and reactive policies cannot keep pace with compound risk. The Valley needs systemic solutions because the problems themselves are systemic.

Once the crisis is understood as solvable, the question shifts from *"Why is this happening?"* to *"Why aren't we fixing it?"*

Why Awareness Alone Is No Longer Enough

Raising awareness is often treated as an end goal. Share the data. Publish the report. Hold the meeting. Post the warning. Then move on.

Awareness matters—but it is only the first step.

The Rio Grande Valley is already aware, at least on a lived level. Residents know the flooding is getting worse. They know water smells different after storms. They know asthma inhalers are common in classrooms. They know cancer diagnoses feel frequent and personal.

What has been missing is not awareness, but **accountability**.

Information without action becomes normalization. When people are repeatedly told that conditions are "within limits" or "being monitored," harm begins to feel unavoidable. Over time, communities adapt to risk rather than demanding its reduction.

This is how environmental injustice becomes permanent.

Awareness must be paired with systems that compel response. Real-time data that triggers intervention. Policies that require cumulative impact analysis. Infrastructure funding tied to risk reduction, not political convenience.

Most importantly, awareness must translate into **public pressure**—pressure that does not fade when the floodwaters recede or the headlines move on.

The Valley does not need more reports that sit on shelves. It needs mechanisms that turn knowledge into change.

The Moral, Economic, and Human Obligation to Act

The obligation to act is not abstract. It is moral, economic, and deeply human.

Morally, no community should accept preventable harm as the cost of living where they were born. Children should not inherit higher disease risk because infrastructure was deferred. Low-income families should not bear disproportionate exposure because they lack political power. These are not unfortunate outcomes—they are ethical failures.

Economically, inaction is irrational.

Every untreated exposure increases healthcare costs. Every flood-damaged home drains household wealth. Every chronically ill worker reduces productivity. Every family that leaves the Valley takes talent, labor, and investment with them.

Environmental neglect is not cheaper. It is simply more expensive later—and paid for by those least able to afford it.

Humanly, the obligation is simplest of all.

People deserve to drink water without wondering what's in it.

They deserve to breathe air without calculating risk.

They deserve homes that are safe from contamination when it rains.

They deserve healthcare systems that are not overwhelmed by preventable disease.

The Rio Grande Valley is home to over a million people. It is not a sacrifice zone. It is not expendable. And it is not too far gone.

But the window to act responsibly is not unlimited.

A Final Call to Action

This book does not end with a prediction. It ends with a choice.

The future of the Rio Grande Valley will be shaped by what happens next—not by what has already happened. The systems described here were built by people. They can be changed by people.

To leaders:

Plan beyond election cycles. Demand cumulative impact assessments. Fund infrastructure where it prevents harm, not where it is most visible. Embrace transparency even when it is uncomfortable. The cost of leadership is responsibility.

CONCLUSION

To institutions and agencies:

Modernize reporting. Share data in real time. Treat communities as partners, not liabilities. Compliance is not the same as protection. Do not confuse minimum standards with sufficient care.

To businesses and developers:

Growth that damages the environment damages the workforce, the market, and the future. Responsible development is not an obstacle—it is an investment in stability.

To healthcare providers and educators:

Continue the work of early detection, education, and advocacy—but do not accept environmental harm as inevitable. Health does not begin in the clinic. It begins in the environment.

To residents:

Your voice matters more than you have been led to believe. Attend meetings. Ask questions. Demand answers. Support policies that protect long-term health over short-term gain. Inaction is not neutrality—it is consent.

And to future generations:

You deserve a Valley that chose to protect itself. You deserve leaders who acted before harm became irreversible. You deserve an environment that supports life rather than eroding it.

The Rio Grande Valley stands at a crossroads.

One path continues the patterns documented in this book—delayed action, fragmented responsibility, and normalized harm. That path leads to higher costs, poorer health, deeper inequality, and fewer choices.

The other path requires courage.

It requires acknowledging uncomfortable truths, investing where it counts, and treating environmental protection as a foundation—not a luxury.

This book has shown what happens when systems are ignored.

The conclusion is simple:

The Valley's future is still being decided.

The only question left is whether we will choose it deliberately—or allow it to be chosen for us.

SOURCES & NOTES

Sources & Notes

This book draws upon publicly available data, peer-reviewed research, investigative journalism, and academic work to examine environmental conditions and public health trends in the Rio Grande Valley. The sources listed below represent the primary references used to inform the analysis, context, and discussion throughout the book.

This section is not exhaustive, but reflects the foundational materials relied upon in good faith.

Regional Environmental & Public Health Data

RGV Health Connect

Regional data platform aggregating public health, environmental, and demographic indicators for the Rio Grande Valley, including air emissions, disease prevalence, and environmental exposure trends.

Data derived from federal and state reporting systems, including EPA and Texas health databases.

Federal Scientific & Environmental Agencies

U.S. Geological Survey (USGS)
Hydrologic, groundwater, watershed, and surface-water studies related to the Rio Grande Basin, Lower Rio Grande Valley, and connected waterways, including water quality, flow patterns, and contaminant transport.

Texas Regulatory & Environmental Agencies

Texas Commission on Environmental Quality (TCEQ)
Water quality assessments, watershed protection plans, impaired water body listings, groundwater monitoring data, Superfund and remediation site documentation, Consumer Confidence Report standards, and environmental permitting records relevant to the Rio Grande Valley.

Investigative Journalism

Inside Climate News
Investigative reporting on environmental infrastructure, wastewater discharges, cross-border pollution, and water quality challenges along the Rio Grande, including documented analysis of sewage releases and regulatory responses.

Academic Research & Theses

The University of Texas Rio Grande Valley (UTRGV)
Graduate theses, faculty research, and academic studies addressing stormwater runoff, land use change, watershed characterization, air quality, public health, and environmental impacts in the Lower Rio Grande Valley.

Peer-Reviewed Scientific Literature

Drinking Water Disinfection Byproducts (DBPs)

Peer-reviewed studies examining the formation of disinfection byproducts, including trihalomethanes (TTHMs) and haloacetic acids (HAA5), and their associations with long-term human health outcomes.

Representative literature includes multidisciplinary reviews published in environmental science and public health journals analyzing epidemiologic evidence, exposure pathways, and regulatory challenges related to DBPs.

Note to Readers

This book does not allege illegal conduct by any individual or entity. It examines documented environmental conditions, publicly reported data, and established scientific research to explore **associations, risks, and systemic challenges** affecting environmental health in the Rio Grande Valley.

Health outcomes discussed are presented at the population level and are not intended as medical or legal advice.

www.ingramcontent.com/pod-product-compliance
Lightning Source LLC
LaVergne TN
LVHW050029080526
838202LV00070B/6975